ERLINDA SABILI

7 Days to Calm:

Doctor-Approved Daily Steps to Reduce Stress, Boost Energy, and Reclaim Your Peace

7 Days to Calm By Dr. Erlinda Asa Sabili, MD, FACP Compassionate Physician & Mental Wellness Advocate As a doctor who's walked the fine line between burnout and balance, I know how hard it is to prioritize your own well-being. But I also know the transformative power of small, intentional practices. In "7 Days to Calm," I'll guide you through daily steps to reduce stress, boost energy, and reclaim your peace. Let's take this journey together, one gentle step at a time.

Contents

Acknowledgments

Writing this book has been a journey of both the heart and mind, and it would not have been possible without the incredible support of so many remarkable individuals.

First and foremost, I extend my deepest gratitude to my family for their unwavering encouragement, patience, and love. Your belief in me gave me the strength to complete this work, even on the most challenging days.

To my colleagues and mentors, thank you for your generosity, expertise, and thoughtful feedback throughout the writing process. Your guidance has helped shape this book into a practical and meaningful resource for readers everywhere.

A special thank you to my editor, Dakie Sabili, and the entire publishing team for clarifying and polishing my words and for your unwavering commitment to excellence.

I would also like to express my heartfelt appreciation to my uncle, Dr. Ben L. Asa; my brother, Attorney Meynard Asa Sabili; and my sisters, Marina Sabili and Marita Sabili Cabatay, for their constant encouragement and support.

My sincere thanks also go to Elizabeth Anne Brown and

to my nieces Bea Marie Sabili Cabatay, Bianca Cabatay, and Bernalyn Cabatay. Your love and inspiration have been an enduring source of strength.

Finally, thank you, the reader, for allowing me to be a part of your journey toward calm and well-being. I hope this book offers you comfort, empowerment, and renewed hope.

Dr. Erlinda Asa Sabili, MD, FACP

Prologue

Why I Wrote This Book
It was a Tuesday morning when I realized something had to change. I had just finished seeing a patient in my outpatient office—a particularly long and emotionally draining one.

I sat in my car, exhausted, with my hands still trembling slightly from the stress of the day. The hospital lights glowed behind me, and the city was just getting ready to sleep. I felt completely exhausted.

I'm both a psychiatrist and an internist. For over two decades, I've had the privilege—and responsibility—of caring for people's minds and bodies. But that evening, I recognized something that's taken me years to admit: I wasn't well either. I was helping everyone else, yet I was silently running on empty.

That moment was a turning point. I began to seek answers not just for my patients but also for myself. I dove deeper into the world of holistic wellness—into mindfulness, movement, nourishing foods, and rituals of rest. And slowly, day by day, I began to heal.

This book is my way of passing along the lifelines that helped me. These are not complex medical treatments or theories tucked away in journals. They are simple, human practices—gentle, evidence-based tools that can change your relationship with stress, one breath at a time.

Why We Need Stress Relief Now—More Than Ever

We live in a world where stress is worn like a badge of honor. We glorify hustle, productivity, and being constantly "on." But what we don't talk about nearly enough is the toll that stress takes on our hearts, hormones, relationships, and joy.

Introduction

7 Days to Calm: Doctor-Approved Daily Steps to Reduce Stress, Boost Energy, and Reclaim Your Peace

7 Days to Calm – A Simple Path to Stress Relief
Stress has become unavoidable in modern life, often lingering in the background like static noise. Though every day, chronic stress is far from harmless—it gradually wears down our energy, disrupts sleep, and contributes to serious health issues like high blood pressure, inflammation, and burnout. As a doctor, I've seen the damage stress can do, but I've also seen how small, intentional daily habits can lead to lasting healing.

That's why I created *7 Days to Calm*—a gentle, practical guide to help you reset your nervous system and restore your inner peace. This isn't about drastic life changes or perfection. Instead, it's about fundamental, practical strategies that fit into your daily routine and spark calm from within.

Through each day of this journey, you explored new ways to calm your nervous system and soothe your busy mind:
    You learned how to use your breath as an anchor—your ever-present tool to return to stillness in any moment.
    You gave your body the gift of gentle movement, releasing tension and inviting balance back in.

You stepped away from the noise by unplugging and decluttering, making space for peace, clarity, and presence.

You embraced the power of micro-meditation, discovering that even a few intentional breaths can reset your day.

You supported your body's natural healing through restful sleep and calming bedtime rituals.

You nourished yourself with foods that heal and strengthen both body and mind.

- Finally, you opened your heart to gratitude—one of the most transformative practices for lasting calm and joy.
-

This journey is about small steps that lead to meaningful transformation. You don't need special equipment or a major lifestyle overhaul—just a willingness to pause, breathe, and care for yourself. Over one week, you'll build a routine that brings more clarity, energy, and calm into your life.

You deserve peace, and I'm honored to guide you there. Welcome to your 7-day calm reset.

Day 1: Breathe Like Your Health Depends On It

Let's start with something you already do—breathe. But today, you'll do it with intention.

As a doctor and someone who has experienced the constant rush of modern life, I can tell you this: one of the most powerful tools for calming stress is already within you—your breath. We breathe every day without thinking—shallow, hurried breaths as we rush from task to task. But that kind of breathing keeps our bodies in a subtle state of stress, reinforcing anxiety and tension.

I used to be skeptical about breathwork. I'd heard all the wellness talk, but I wondered *if breathing could change anything.* But after years of using breath techniques and teaching them to patients, I've seen how something so simple can shift your entire state of being. Breath is your body's built-in reset button—free, always available, and incredibly effective.

The Science Behind It

When we're stressed, our sympathetic nervous system kicks in—what's known as the fight-or-flight mode. This can be useful in emergencies, but it's harmful when it's always on. Deep, intentional breathing flips that switch. It activates the parasympathetic nervous system, which helps us rest, digest, and heal.

Just 2–5 minutes of deep breathing can lower cortisol (your stress hormone), slow your heart rate, calm your mind, and help you feel grounded again. It can improve your sleep, focus, and energy. It's one of the simplest ways to bring your body back into balance.

Try This Now: The Calm Breathing Exercise

1. Sit or lie down comfortably.
2. Place one hand on your belly and the other on your chest.
3. Inhale slowly through your nose for a count of 4.
4. Hold your breath gently for 2 seconds.
5. Exhale slowly through your mouth for a count of 6.
6. Repeat for 5–10 breaths.

Feel your belly rise as you inhale and fall as you exhale. That belly movement is a good sign—you're breathing deeply, not just into your chest.

Optional: Box Breathing

Used by Navy Seals and elite athletes, this technique quickly calms the nervous system:

- Inhale for four counts
- Hold for four counts
- Exhale for four counts

- Hold for four counts
- Repeat 3–4 rounds.

When to Use This

- Before a stressful meeting
- During moments of anxiety
- As part of your bedtime wind-down
- First thing in the morning
- Anytime you need a reset.

Make It Personal

Anchor this practice to something you already do—your morning coffee, brushing your teeth, or winding down for bed. You can even pair it with calming music for a more profound effect (there's a curated playlist in the bonus section of the book).

Your Day 1 Challenge

Today, take five minutes to practice calm breathing. Set a timer, find a quiet spot, and breathe. Later, reflect on how you felt before and after. Where do you carry stress in your body? How can you remind yourself to return to your breath tomorrow?

Remember: one breath won't change everything, but consistent practice will. This is your first step toward calm. You're doing something powerful and healing, and I'm right here with you. Let's breathe.

Do the Meditation on Evening Calmness in Dr. Erlinda Sabili's List of Healing Harmony. Scan the QR code on the back with your smartphone, or check my YouTube channel @lindasabili1051 under Lyrical Dreams.

Day 2: Move Gently Move your Body Calm your Mind

Today's goal isn't a workout—it's movement that feels *good* in your body. Not the kind that pushes or punishes, but the kind that soothes, nourishes, and brings you home to yourself.

In a world that constantly glorifies hustle and high-intensity exercise, it's easy to forget that gentle, intentional movement can be just as powerful, especially when managing stress and lifting one's mood. Movement can shift one's energy and settle one's nervous system, whether it's a slow walk in the park, stretching on one's living room floor, or swaying to one's favorite song in the kitchen.

Why Gentle Movement Matters

When you move, even slowly, your body releases endorphins—those natural chemicals that help you feel better. It also improves circulation, clears away excess cortisol (the stress hormone), and helps regulate your mood. You don't need a gym membership or a fancy routine. You must tune in and ask your body what would feel good right now.

Gentle movement also improves sleep, supports your immune system, and restores a sense of calm. It helps you come back into your body, especially when anxiety or overwhelm pull you into your head.

What Movement Could Look Like Today

The beauty of this practice is its simplicity. Choose one or more of the following, and aim for about 10–20 minutes, or whatever feels right:

- Take a Slow Walk Outdoors
- Let your walk be about presence, not pace. Leave your phone behind, take in your surroundings, breathe deeply, and notice the rhythm of your steps.
- Stretch on the Floor
- Try gentle yoga poses like Child's Pose, Cat-Cow, or Forward Fold. These help release tension in common stress spots like the neck, shoulders, and hips.
- Dance in Your Living Room
- Put on a favorite song and let your body move freely—no choreography, no rules—just joy.
- Movement Meditation
- Try slowly rotating your wrists, shoulders, and ankles with full awareness. Feel each joint awaken.
- Bedside Routine
- Stretch gently when you wake or before bed—arms overhead, gentle twists, or raising your legs to support circulation.

Tips for Success

- Set the Mood: Light a candle, play calming music, or open a window. Make it a moment, not a chore.
- Let Go of Rules: This is not about reps, routines, or results. It's about reconnecting.
- Listen In: Ask, *"What would feel good to my body right now?"* Then honor that answer.

Doctor's Perspective

In my years working with patients, I've witnessed how even small amounts of movement—like a short walk down a hospital hallway—can lift a person's spirit, ease anxiety, and reignite hope. You don't need to be recovering from an illness to experience the healing power of movement. You need to begin.

Today's Challenge

Move gently for at least 10 minutes. Let it feel light, kind, and true to you. Then pause, close your eyes, and notice: *How does my body feel now compared to before?* This is how we return to ourselves—one breath, step, and stretch at a time.

Remember: movement is medicine; today, your body is the pharmacy.

Use the guided meditation, Lunch Break Relaxation Meditation.

Do the Meditation on Lunch Break Relaxation Meditation found in the List of Healing Harmony by Dr.Erlinda Sabili. Scan the QR code on the back of your smartphone or check my YouTube channel @lindasabili1051 under Lyrical Dreams. Day 2: Move Your Body, Calm Your Mind

Day 3 : Unplug and Declutter for Inner Peace

Today, I invite you to do something both incredibly simple and surprisingly powerful: step away from your screens. Even if it's just for one hour, it could make a real difference in how your mind and body feel.

Let's be honest—most of us have way too many tabs open, both on our devices and in our minds. Between social media, emails, news updates, and constant notifications, we're bombarded with information all day long. It's no wonder we often feel anxious, scattered, or mentally drained. Our brains were never designed to process this much input at once, and yet we rarely give them time to rest.

That's where today's practice comes in. I call it *Digital Detox Lite*. No, you don't have to give up technology completely or disappear into the woods. But for just one hour today, power down. Turn off your phone, close the laptop, step away from the TV—and reconnect with yourself.

Your Challenge:

Schedule one hour without any screens. Use this time to do something restorative:

- Take a walk outside and listen to the wind or the birds.
- Journal what's on your mind or reflect on your day.
- Read a physical book or magazine.
- Cook something slowly and mindfully.
- Or just rest, without trying to be productive.

The goal isn't to be "better" or "more efficient." The goal is space—mental and emotional space. And in that space, something beautiful happens. Your breath naturally deepens. Your heart rate slows. Your mind begins to quiet. You begin to feel—maybe for the first time all day—that you're actually *here*, not pulled in a hundred directions.

When I first tried this, I didn't expect much. I figured an hour away from screens wouldn't change anything. But what I found surprised me: I felt calmer, more centered, more like *me*. It was like hitting the reset button on a day that had felt too fast, too full, and too loud.

Even more, stepping away from screens before bed can improve your sleep, help you unwind, and ease tension you didn't even know you were holding. Try making your bedroom a "no phone zone" or lighting a candle instead of scrolling before sleep. Small changes like these send your nervous system a powerful message: It's okay to rest. You're safe now.

Pro tip: If your mind is racing, grab a notebook and do a quick "brain dump." Write down everything swirling around—your to-dos, your worries, your random thoughts. Seeing them on paper can bring instant relief, like clearing out mental clutter.

So today, give yourself this gift: one hour of peace. No buzzing, no pings, no updates. Just you, your breath, and the quiet. Let your nervous system exhale. You don't need to earn rest. You deserve it.

Your peace is waiting—it just needs a little space to rise.

Let's Meditate using Meditation Letting Go with Dr. Erlinda Sabili found in the List of Healing Harmony by Dr.Erlinda Sabili. Scan the QR code at the back with your smartphone or check my YouTube channel @lindasabili1051 under Lyrical dreams.

Day 4:Master the Art of Micro-Meditation

Today's invitation is simple: slow down and *breathe*. That's it. You don't need a mountaintop, a meditation cushion, or 30 minutes of silence. You just need *two minutes*—maybe even less. Welcome to the gentle art of micro-meditation.

Contrary to popular belief, meditation isn't about having a blank mind. It's not about "doing it right" or achieving enlightenment. It's simply about returning to the present moment. And in that return, something magical happens—your breath slows, your thoughts settle, and your nervous system softens. Even one intentional breath can make a difference.
Let me share a simple meditation practice from a doctor who uses it with patients in hospitals, especially during stressful moments:

1. Sit comfortably—on a chair, your bed, or the floor.
2. Close your eyes, or gently lower your gaze.
3. Breathe in slowly, saying to yourself: *"Inhale calm."*
4. Breathe out slowly, saying: *"Exhale tension."*
5. When your mind wanders (and it will), gently come back

to the breath.
6. Continue for 2–5 minutes.

That's it. No pressure. No need to be perfect. Just be present.

But here's the beautiful thing—you don't have to set aside special time in your day to feel the benefits of mindfulness. Micro-meditation is about sprinkling short, grounding moments into your life, wherever you are. It's like sipping water instead of chugging a whole glass. Small, consistent sips of calm.

Here's a quick 2-minute mindfulness routine you can do anytime:

- Step 1: Body Scan (40 seconds)
- Gently bring your attention to your body—starting with your feet and slowly moving upward. Notice sensations, tension, or warmth. You don't need to change anything. Just observe.
- Step 2: Breathing (40 seconds)
- Turn your focus to your breath. Inhale deeply, exhale softly. Notice the rise and fall of your chest or the cool air through your nose.
- Step 3: Gratitude (40 seconds)
- Think of one thing you're grateful for—just one. A person, a pet, a meal, or even your breath. Let that feeling of appreciation sink in.

You just meditated. And your body and mind are already thanking you.

Let's also debunk a few common myths:

16

- Myth 1: "I need to clear my mind."
- Not true. Your mind *will* wander. The goal is not to stop thinking, but to notice when your attention drifts and gently return to the breath. That gentle return *is* the practice.
- Myth 2: "I'm doing it wrong if I get distracted."
- Distraction is part of the process. Every time you notice it and come back—you're building awareness and resilience.
- Myth 3: "I don't have time."
- You do. One breath. One moment. One pause in your day is enough to reset.

So today, I encourage you to carve out a few moments of stillness. It could be in the car before you drive, at your desk between tasks, or while your tea steeps. You don't need anything but *yourself*.

Peace is only ever a breath away.

Day 5: The Power of Sleep Hygiene

Day 5: The Power of Sleep Hygiene

Why Better Sleep is the Key to a Calmer, Healthier You

Let's be real—when life gets overwhelming, sleep is usually the first thing to go. We stay up late, scroll through our phones in bed, and then wonder why we feel drained, foggy, or short-tempered the next day. But sleep isn't a luxury—it's essential. It's the body's natural repair system, and when we don't get enough of it, everything suffers: our patience, our focus, our immunity, and even our emotional balance.

Stress and poor sleep are deeply connected. When you're under pressure, your body kicks into "fight or flight" mode, releasing stress hormones like cortisol. That's okay in small doses, but if it becomes chronic, cortisol fuels inflammation—the kind that's linked to heart disease, anxiety, depression, and autoimmune conditions. And what feeds that inflammation even more? Yep—bad sleep. It's a vicious cycle:

Stress → Less Sleep → More Inflammation → More Stress

Breaking this loop doesn't require a complete life overhaul. It starts with small, intentional shifts in your nightly routine— what doctors call *sleep hygiene*. This means designing your habits and environment to support deeper, more restorative rest. Think of it as a way to gently tell your body, *"You're safe now. It's okay to let go."*

☽ Doctor's 5-Step Bedtime Ritual

These simple practices can help calm your mind, lower stress, and set the stage for quality sleep:

✔ 1. **Unplug One Hour Before Bed**

Turn off screens and dim the lights. Blue light from phones, tablets, and TVs blocks melatonin—the hormone that helps you fall asleep. Instead, unwind with journaling, reading, or soft music.

✔ 2. **Practice a 2-Minute Wind-Down**

Breathe deeply. Try a short body scan or silently repeat, *"I am safe. I am calm."* Even two minutes of stillness tells your nervous system the day is done.

✔ 3. **Sip Something Soothing**

Try chamomile tea, warm almond milk, or turmeric "golden milk." These herbal drinks are calming and naturally anti-inflammatory. Skip caffeine, alcohol, and heavy meals in the evening.

✔ 4. **Set the Scene for Sleep**

Keep your bedroom cool, dark, and quiet. Use blackout curtains, an eye mask, or a white noise machine. Make the space feel peaceful—like a cocoon, not a workspace.

✔ 5. **Stick to a Consistent Sleep-Wake Schedule**

Go to bed and wake up at the same time each day—even on weekends. This trains your internal clock and helps you fall asleep faster and wake up refreshed.

Tonight's Challenge

Try the 5-step ritual tonight. Even doing just one or two steps sends a clear message to your body: *It's safe to rest.* If you wake up in the night, don't reach for your phone. Instead, place one hand on your chest, the other on your belly, and breathe slowly. Let your breath guide you back to sleep.

✫ Final Thought

Sleep is your body's way of healing and restoring. It quiets the stress, soothes inflammation, and strengthens your emotional resilience. You don't need to fix everything overnight—just begin. A little intention, a little calm, and a whole lot of self-kindness can change everything. You deserve that kind of rest.

Day 6: Nourish Your Body Eat to Beat Stress

Let's talk about food—not as calories or macros, but as *messages*. Every bite we take sends a signal to the body: *You're safe... or you're stressed.* That's right—food is more than fuel. It's communication. And especially in stressful times, what we eat can either soothe or stir our nervous system.

We've all been there: overwhelmed, anxious, or exhausted, and suddenly that bag of chips or extra coffee feels like comfort. And honestly? That's human. There's no shame in those cravings— they're often just a signal that our body is crying out for stability. The challenge is that those quick fixes (like sugar, caffeine, or processed snacks) might feel good in the moment, but they actually add to our body's stress load. They can spike blood sugar, increase inflammation, and leave us feeling even more frazzled.

Here's the good news: your plate can be part of your healing.

🌿 *What to Focus On: Stress-Soothing Nutrition*

Start by adding more of these:

- Whole, colorful fruits and vegetables – These are rich in antioxidants, which help fight the damage that chronic stress does to your body.
- Healthy fats – Think avocado, olive oil, chia seeds, and nuts. These support brain function and reduce inflammation.
- Hydration – Dehydration can actually mimic anxiety. So, keep that water bottle nearby!
- Calming teas – Chamomile, peppermint, and rooibos are gentle ways to relax your body and mind.

🔥 *The Inflammation Connection*

Chronic stress leads to chronic inflammation—a silent contributor to everything from heart disease to depression. But here's where food becomes medicine: anti-inflammatory choices like berries, leafy greens, turmeric, and omega-3-rich foods (like salmon and walnuts) can help your body return to balance.

Eating well isn't about being perfect—it's about creating *calm from the inside out.*

🧘‍♀️ *Eat to Calm Your Nervous System*

Certain nutrients are especially good for stress relief:

- Magnesium (found in leafy greens, seeds, and dark chocolate) helps relax muscles and calm the mind.

- Omega-3s (from fatty fish, flaxseeds, and walnuts) support brain health and reduce anxiety.
- Antioxidants (from fruits and vegetables) protect your cells from stress-related damage.

Even one nourishing choice a day can make a difference. Try a simple smoothie, a cozy homemade soup, or even just swap your third coffee for a herbal tea.

🍵 Try This Calming Smoothie:

- 1 banana
- A handful of spinach
- 1 tablespoon almond butter
- 1 cup unsweetened almond milk
- Ice

Blend and enjoy. It's rich in magnesium, fiber, and healthy fats—a mini hug in a glass.

Final Thought:
Food doesn't have to be complicated to be healing. Every small, loving choice you make—adding greens to your plate, sipping a calming tea, or drinking more water—is an act of self-care. You're not just feeding your body; you're telling yourself: *I matter. I'm worth slowing down for.*
Today's challenge? Make one nourishing choice. That's it. Your body—and your nervous system—will thank you.
Have a relaxing day using Let's Meditate with Dr. Erlinda Sabili

found in the List of Healing Harmony by Dr.Erlinda Sabili. Scan the QR code at the back with your smartphone or check my YouTube channel @lindasabili1051 under Lyrical dreams.

Day 7: Gratitude + The Doctor's Joy Reset

Day 7: Gratitude + The Doctor's Joy Reset

You Did It! A Gentle Celebration of Calm, Gratitude, and Growth

Pause for a moment. Please close your eyes, take a slow, deep breath in… and let it go. Feel that? That's the calm you've been creating, one breath, one intention, one gentle step at a time.

Congratulations—you've completed the *7 Days to Calm* challenge! Whether you followed it perfectly or showed up in the best way you could each day, you've done something meaningful for your mind, body, and spirit. That deserves acknowledgment and celebration.

One of the most powerful takeaways from this journey is the practice of *gratitude*. It's more than just saying "thank you"—it's a scientifically backed way to *rewire* your brain and help your body find balance. Research shows that practicing gratitude can:

- Lower your stress hormone (cortisol)
- Decrease symptoms of anxiety and depression.
- Boost serotonin and dopamine—the brain's "feel good" chemicals.
- Improve sleep, immune function, and emotional resiliency

Gratitude gently shifts your perspective—from what's missing or stressful to what is *already present and good*. And that shift can be life-changing. Especially when life feels overwhelming, this small, consistent habit can serve as your anchor.

Your Gratitude Journal Starter

You don't need to write an essay or have the perfect words. Gratitude blooms in simplicity. Use this gentle journalism prompt any time—morning, night, or in between:

- **Today I'm grateful for...**
- **Something small that made me smile today:**
- **A challenge I faced—and one thing I learned from it:**
- **One person I appreciate and why:**

Remember, if you're ever unsure what to write, start with the basics: a roof over your head, warm food, someone who listens, or simply a peaceful moment. Gratitude isn't about grand gestures—it's about noticing the beauty in the everyday.

You've Built a Toolkit for Life

Let's look back on what you've embraced over the past seven days:

- Breath work to calm your nervous system and anchor yourself in the present
   - Gentle movement to release tension and reconnect with your body
   - Unplugging and decluttering to clear space and simplify your surroundings
   - Micro-meditation to reset your mind and reframe your thoughts with kindness
   - Evening rituals to improve your sleep and restore your energy
   - Mindful nourishment to care for your body with love and intention
   - And finally, gratitude, to bring joy and peace into your daily life

These aren't just tips—they're tools. And now they're yours. You can return to them repeatedly, like trusted friends, whenever you need to re-center. This isn't about perfection—it's about progress. About coming back to yourself, gently, day by day.

Where Do You Go From Here

This challenge was your *first step*, not your final destination. Calm is a journey, not a finish line. You've begun healing and reconnecting with your inner peace—and that's a journey worth continuing.

Be kind to yourself. Some days will feel easier than others. That's okay. What matters is that you keep choosing yourself. Keep choosing peace. Keep choosing to notice the good, even in small, quiet ways.

Final Reflections and Invitation

♈ **Challenge:** Write down three things you're grateful for today.

💡 **Doctor's Tip:** Start or end your day with gratitude to create a sense of calm and clarity.

Reflection: Has your mindset or mood shifted through this practice? What have you discovered about yourself?

As you continue your path forward, know this: you are capable. You are resilient. And you are worthy of the peace you're creating.

Thank you for showing up for yourself. Keep breathing, keep going, and keep noticing the light, even on cloudy days.

With heartfelt gratitude,

Dr. Erlinda Asa Sabili, MD, FACP

Bonus Resource Library: Meditations & Songs for Calm and Wellness

As a special companion to *7 Days to Calm*, I'm excited to share a collection of my original guided meditations, songs, and exercise tracks designed to deepen your healing journey.

These free resources are available anytime to help you breathe easier, calm your mind, move your body, and lift your spirit. Visit the following links or scan the QR code on this page to access the audio library.

🎧 *1. Guided Meditations*

- Let's Meditate
- Evening Calmness
- Lunch Break Relaxation Meditation
- Morning Calmness
- Coping with Loss: A Guided Meditation for Grief
- Meditation: Letting Go
- Meditation on Life's Uncertainty
- Message About Growing Old

♪ 2. Worship and Love Songs

- Hope in Our Hearts
- A Love that Lasts
- Slipping Away
- Love That Remains
- Love Is The Way
- Love Is The Answer
- Growing Old with Grace
- Love Notes from God
- Love's Embrace
- Reach Out
- Healing Hands
- Lord, Teach Me How to Pray
- Make Me One with You
- Cheerfulness of God
- Love and Forgiveness
- Watching Over Me
- You Are Not Alone
- Pilgrims of Hope
- God's Love Forever Stands
- Grandma's Baking Battle
- Grandparents' Love

♪♪ 3. Exercise & Movement Songs

- Step by Step
- Get Moving, Stay Grooving
- Get Moving
- Sweat and Smile
- Fitness Frenzy

- God's Got Our Back
- Healthy Habits
- Unstoppable
- Move Your Body

I hope these meditations and songs are a trusted companion on your journey toward calm, wellness, and joy.
Dr. Erlinda Asa Sabili

About 7 Days to Calm

In a world that moves faster than ever, 7 Days to Calm allows you to pause, breathe, and rediscover balance.

This doctor-approved guide was created for busy people like you: caregivers, healthcare professionals, parents, and anyone longing for peace amid life's chaos.

Dr. Erlinda Asa Sabili—a physician, psychiatrist, and passionate advocate for holistic wellness—shares her proven 7-step method to help you reduce stress, boost energy, and reclaim your sense of calm.

You'll learn:

- How to use your breath as an anchor in stressful moments
- How gentle movement restores harmony between body and mind
- The power of decluttering, micro-meditation, and restful sleep
- How nutrition and gratitude practices build lasting resilience

Whether you revisit the program repeatedly or simply integrate pieces of it into your daily life, *7 Days to Calm* is your personal prescription for peace.

For more guided meditations, original music, and resources to support your calm journey, visit: Healing Harmony

Conclusion

Dear Friend,

Congratulations. Truly—from the bottom of my heart, congratulations. You've completed the *7 Days to Calm* challenge, deeply worth celebrating. In a world that often rushes past our needs, that tells us to do more, be more, fix more, you choose to slow down. You decided to breathe. You chose to care for yourself.

I hope you let that sink in. Because it takes courage to pause, it takes strength to turn inward, to gently peel back the layers of stress and overwhelm and reconnect with yourself. That's what you've done this past week—step by step, breath by breath. You didn't just go through the motions. You showed up for yourself in a powerful, beautiful way.

You may not feel completely different right now. That's okay. Transformation doesn't always shout. Sometimes, it whispers. Sometimes, it arrives in subtle shifts—in how you speak to yourself, how your shoulders soften, and how you pause before reacting. But know this: something *has* shifted. You planted seeds this week, and they *will* grow.

This is just the beginning.

Healing and calm aren't destinations—they are practices. Ongoing, living, breathing experiences. So don't worry if you didn't do it "perfectly." Life isn't a performance. It's a process. And you've already taken the most essential step: *beginning*. That alone is something so many people struggle with, and you did it.

I invite you to **return to this challenge anytime**. Make it a monthly ritual, a reset button whenever life feels heavy. You can revisit your favorite day or re-explore each step in a new way. Some parts may feel easier next time. Others may surprise you. That's the beauty of this work—it meets you exactly where you are.

If you found this journey helpful, please consider **sharing it**. We all know someone who carries invisible weight—stress, anxiety, grief, burnout. You now have a roadmap that might help them breathe a little easier, too. Your calm is not just your gift—it can become your legacy, rippling outward in ways you may never fully see.

To support you even further, I've created **free calming tools** just for you. On my website, you'll find soothing guided meditations, music playlists to unwind, breathing exercises, and mindfulness resources to help you deepen the calm you've begun to cultivate. Think of it as your digital sanctuary—a peaceful place to return anytime.

☞ Visit here: Healing Harmony

You might also enjoy my other books and offerings, which

explore themes of emotional healing, mindful living, better sleep, and self-compassion. My mission is simple: to help you reconnect with the most peaceful, grounded version of yourself. You *deserve* that version.

Before you close this chapter, I encourage you to pause for a moment.

Place your hand over your heart.

Take a slow, deep breath in.

And as you exhale, silently say to yourself: *"I am proud of how far I've come."*

Because you should be.

You have tended to your inner world in a way that few people ever do. You've reminded yourself that you are *not your stress.* You are not your mistakes, anxiety, or to-do list you haven't finished. You are so much more.

You are a human being with a heart that wants to heal and a mind that wants peace.

Keep choosing calm, even in small ways. Write down three things you're grateful for. Stretch your body. Step outside and feel the sun. Breathe deeply. Smile at something simple.

Let this become a part of who you are—not just something you *do*, but something you *live*.

Let's be honest: the world will still be busy. Life will still have its waves. But now you have tools. You have awareness. And you have a quiet strength that's been awakened.

This is your journey. Walk it gently. Walk it boldly. Walk it with love.

With deep gratitude and peace,

CONCLUSION

Dr. Erlinda Asa Sabili, MD, FACP

Resources and References

The following resources and references have informed and inspired the guidance provided in 7 Days to Calm. While this book is intended as a practical companion, readers seeking further knowledge and scientific insight may find these materials helpful. Additional resources include recommended reading, scientific articles, and online tools.

- American Psychological Association. (2020). Publication manual of the American Psychological Association (7th ed.). American Psychological Association.

- Brewer, J. A. (2021). Unwinding anxiety: New science shows how to break the cycles of worry and fear to heal your mind. Avery.

- Kabat-Zinn, J. (2013). Full catastrophe living: Using the wisdom of your body and mind to face stress, pain, and illness (Revised ed.). Bantam.

- Neff, K. (2011). Self-compassion: The proven power of being kind to yourself. William Morrow.

- Siegel, D. J. (2010). Mindsight: The new science of personal transformation. Bantam Books.

- Sabili, E. A. (2025). 7 Days to Calm: Doctor-Approved Daily Steps to Reduce Stress, Boost Energy, and Reclaim Your Peace.

- Davidson, R. J., & Begley, S. (2012). The emotional life of your brain: How its unique patterns affect the way you think, feel, and live-and how you can change them. Hudson Street Press.

- Goleman, D. (2011). The brain and emotional intelligence: New insights. More Than Sound.
- Hanson, R. (2013). Hardwiring happiness: The new brain science of contentment, calm, and confidence. Harmony.

- Maté, G. (2019). When the body says no: Exploring the stress-disease connection. Vintage Canada.

- Van der Kolk, B. A. (2014). The body keeps the score: Brain, mind, and body in the healing of trauma. Viking.

- Brown, B. (2018). Dare to lead: Brave work. Tough conversations. Whole hearts. Random House.

- Dweck, C. S. (2006). Mindset: The new psychology of success. Random House.

Gawande, A. (2014). Being mortal: Medicine and what matters in the end. Metropolitan Books.

- Linehan, M. M. (2014). DBT skills training manual (2nd ed.). Guilford Press.Tolle, E. (2005). A new earth: Awakening to your life's purpose. Penguin Group.

- Williams, M., Teasdale, J., Segal, Z., & Kabat-Zinn, J. (2007). The mindful way through depression: Freeing yourself from chronic unhappiness. Guilford Press.

- Porges, S. W. (2017). The pocket guide to the polyvagal theory: The transformative power of feeling safe. W. W. Norton & Company.

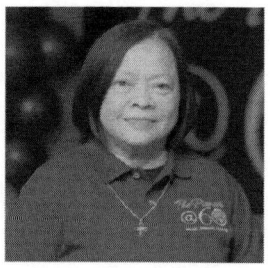

About the Author

About Dr. Erlinda Asa Sabili

Dr. Erlinda Asa Sabili, MD, FACP, is a compassionate physician who bridges the worlds of internal medicine, psychiatry, and theology to offer a holistic approach to healing. With over two decades of experience, she has dedicated her career to helping individuals find balance and peace in their lives.

Dr. Sabili believes that true wellness encompasses both the body and the mind. Her unique integration of medical science and spiritual insight allows her to address the whole person, not just symptoms. She is passionate about empowering people with practical strategies to take control of their health and well-being.

Beyond her medical practice, Dr. Sabili is a creative soul who finds joy in composing songs and meditations. Through her book, 7 Days to Calm, she shares her insights and tools to help readers reduce stress and cultivate lasting peace.

You can connect with me on:

f https://www.facebook.com/linda.sabili.5

⌘ https://www.youtube.com/@lindasabili1051

Made in the USA
Monee, IL
30 June 2025

20317335R00028